MASTERING MINDSET FOR FITNESS SUCCESS

MASTERING MINDSET FOR FITNESS SUCCESS

TECHNIQUES FOR CULTIVATING A POSITIVE MINDSET THAT SUPPORTS FITNESS GOALS

ADAM FRASER

VISIONS AND VOICES
TULSA, OKLAHOMA

Mastering Mindset for Fitness Success
Adam Fraser
Visions and Voices
Copyright © 2024
Cataloging information
ISBN-13 979-8327229990

DEDICATION

To my children,

This book, "Mastering Mindset for Fitness Success," is lovingly dedicated to you. Your unwavering support, belief in my potential, and endless encouragement have been the foundation upon which this journey was built. In moments of doubt, it was your faith that shone like a beacon, guiding me back to my path with a renewed sense of purpose and determination.

Your presence in my life has been a profound source of inspiration. Watching you grow, embrace challenges with bravery, and navigate the world with curiosity and kindness has taught me more about resilience, love, and the power of a positive mindset than any book or experience ever could. You have unwittingly become my teachers, showing me the importance of pursuing one's passions with heart and dedication.

As you leaf through these pages, know that it is not just a book about fitness and mindset but a narrative that has been profoundly influenced by your spirits and characters. It is my deepest hope that this book not only serves as a guide for others on their fitness journeys but also as a reminder to you of the incredible impact you have on those around you.

To my children, thank you for your love, your support, and for believing in me even when I struggled to believe in myself. Your confidence in my abilities has been a driving force behind this endeavor, pushing me to strive for excellence and to make a difference in the lives of others. As this book finds its way into the hands of readers, let it also serve as a symbol of my gratitude and love for you.

May we continue to inspire each other, grow together, and face life's challenges with the same courage and positivity that you have shown me. This dedication, and indeed this book, is for you—a small token of my immense love and appreciation.

—Adam

ACKNOWLEDGEMENTS

I would like to express my deepest gratitude to everyone who played a part in the realization of this book. Special thanks to Mary Van Orman, for her invaluable advice and encouragement, and to my children, whose support and patience were my anchors. To the many in the fitness and psychology community who shared their insights, thank you for enriching this work with your expertise.

FOREWARD

In this life, we are often told that the path to success is linear—that if we just follow a set of steps, success is guaranteed. But anyone who has truly pursued a dream, faced down challenges, or sought to make a lasting change knows that the journey is anything but straightforward. It's a path filled with setbacks, learning, and, most importantly, growth. This is why Adam Fraser's "Mastering Mindset for Fitness Success" is not just a book; it's a roadmap to understanding that the most crucial battles on the way to achieving our fitness goals, and indeed any goals, are fought in the mind.

I've had the privilege of working with Adam and experiencing his holistic approach to fitness. It's not just about the physical transformation—which is, without doubt, remarkable—but about the mental and emotional resilience that his training instills. This book encapsulates that philosophy, offering not just strategies and techniques but a way to reframe your entire approach to fitness and wellness.

Adam understands something that I've tried to embody in my own life and work: that stories have power. The narratives we tell ourselves about who we are, what we're capable of, and what we can overcome are foundational to our success. "Mastering Mindset for Fitness Success" invites you to consider your own story, challenging you to rewrite the limiting beliefs that hold you back and embrace a mindset of growth and possibility.

Reading through these pages, you're not just learning how to set goals or stick to a workout routine; you're learning how to cultivate a mindset that will empower you in every area of your life. Adam's approach to fitness is a metaphor for overcoming challenges, facing fears, and pushing beyond what we thought was possible. It's about the transformation that begins in the heart and mind, long before it's visible on the outside.

To those picking up this book, whether you're at the start of your fitness journey or looking to deepen your practice, know this: you hold in your hands not just a guide to physical fitness but a manual for transforming your life. The principles Adam shares are those I've seen him live by—principles that have inspired me in dark times and that I know can inspire you, too.

Embrace this journey with an open heart and mind. Let Adam's wisdom guide you, not just on the path to physical wellness, but towards a life lived with purpose, resilience, and unshakeable belief in your own potential. Here's to your success, on and off the fitness floor.

—Tyler Perry

PREFACE

In the journey of writing "Mastering Mindset for Fitness Success," my aim was to illuminate the oft-underestimated role of mindset in the pursuit of fitness goals. This book is born out of a combination of personal experience, extensive research, and countless conversations with fitness professionals and enthusiasts alike. It is designed to guide you through the mental and emotional landscapes that are as much a part of achieving fitness success as the physical aspect.

Herein, you'll find not just strategies and techniques but stories of real individuals who have transformed their lives through the principles discussed in these pages. My hope is that their journeys will inspire you, as they have inspired me, to believe in the possibility of change and the power of a positive mindset.

INTRODUCTION

Welcome to "Mastering Mindset for Fitness Success," where your journey to achieving and surpassing your fitness goals begins not with a step, but with a thought. This book is designed to challenge and change how you think about fitness, success, and the role of mindset in bridging the two.

The road to fitness success is often paved with misconceptions that it's all about willpower, routine, or the perfect diet. While these elements play a role, they are but pieces of a larger puzzle. The missing piece, and the focus of this book, is the mindset. Without the right mindset, sustaining motivation, overcoming obstacles, and achieving long-term success becomes an uphill battle.

Through the forthcoming chapters, we will dissect the elements of a powerful fitness mindset, from setting achievable goals and overcoming obstacles to building lasting habits and staying motivated. Each section is filled with actionable advice, grounded in the latest psychological research and illustrated with inspiring success stories.

This book is not just about reading; it's about action. It's about transforming the way you think about fitness from a temporary endeavor to a lifelong journey of growth and fulfillment. So, as you turn these pages, I encourage you to engage actively with the exercises, reflect on the insights, and apply the strategies to your own life.

Let's embark on this transformative journey together. Your fitness success story starts now.

TABLE OF CONTENTS

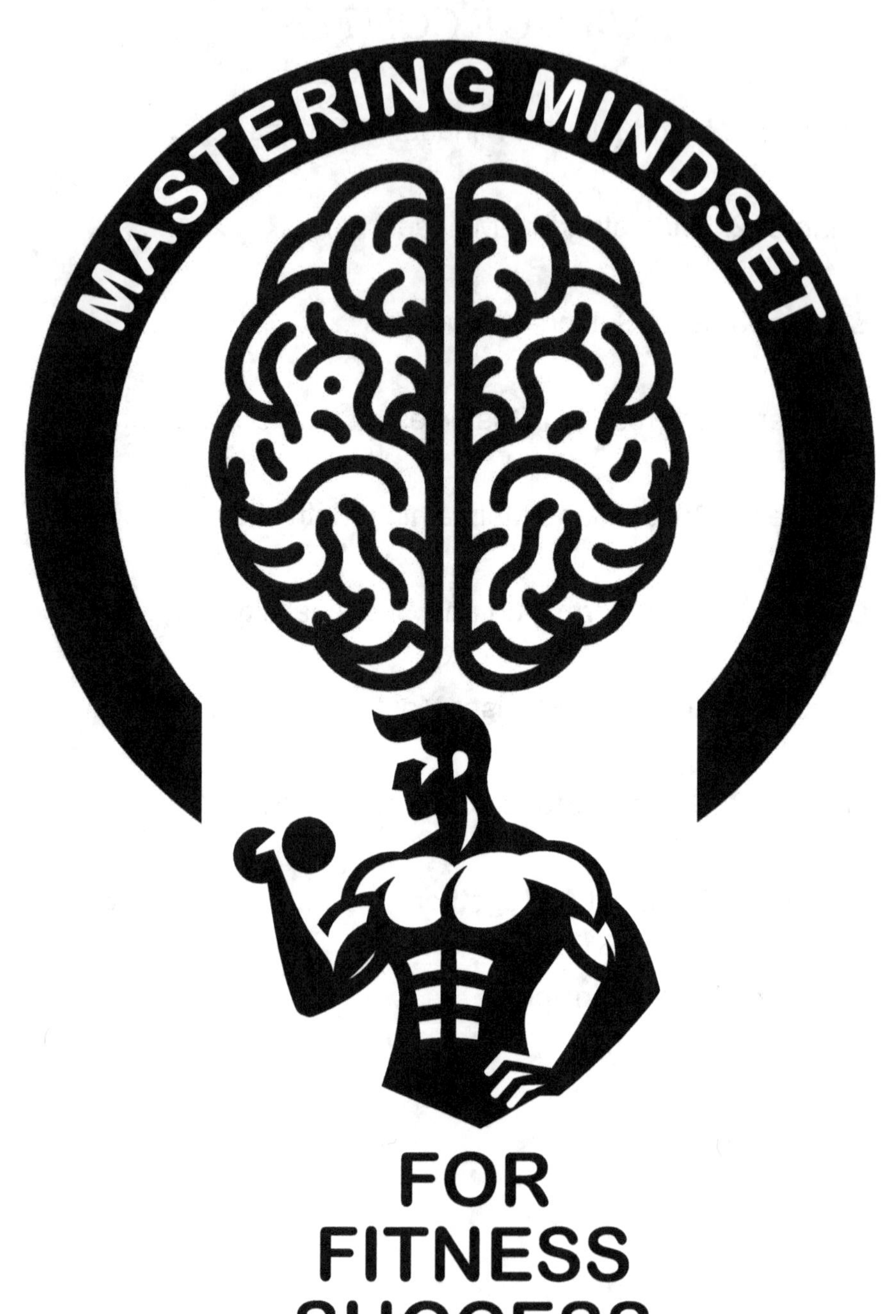
MASTERING MINDSET
FOR
FITNESS
SUCCESS

CHAPTER 1: INTRODUCTION TO MINDSET IN FITNESS

The Foundation of Fitness Success

Welcome to "Mastering Mindset for Fitness Success," where we embark on a transformative journey to understand the profound impact of mindset on achieving and sustaining fitness goals. Fitness is not solely a physical endeavor; it is equally a mental challenge. The journey to improved health and fitness begins in the mind. Before we delve into strategies, techniques, and inspirational stories, it's crucial to establish why mindset matters in fitness.

The Role of Mindset in Fitness

Mindset, the collection of beliefs and attitudes that shape how we interpret and interact with the world, is the cornerstone of every fitness journey. It influences our motivation, resilience, and willingness to embrace challenges. A positive mindset can be the difference between success and setback, pushing us to overcome obstacles and persevere in the face of adversity.

Understanding the role of mindset in fitness involves recognizing two fundamental truths:

1. **Physical actions are guided by mental beliefs:** How we perceive our abilities and our fitness goals deeply influences our commitment to them. Believing in our capacity to change and grow (a growth mindset) leads to more sustained effort and resilience compared to seeing our abilities as fixed and unchangeable.

2. **Mindset shapes our response to challenges:** Encountering obstacles is inevitable on any fitness journey. A positive mindset equips us with the strategies to view these challenges as opportunities for growth rather than insurmountable barriers.

Objective of This Book

The primary goal of this Book is to guide you through the process of cultivating a positive mindset that not only supports but amplifies your fitness goals. Through the pages that follow, you will learn how to:

- Set and achieve realistic fitness goals.

- Overcome common psychological and physical barriers.

- Maintain motivation and commitment to your fitness journey.

- Form and sustain habits that support your fitness objectives.

- Utilize advanced mindset techniques to continuously improve your fitness and overall well-being.

What to Expect

As we progress through each chapter, we will explore the intricacies of the fitness mindset, from setting the foundation in goal-setting strategies to overcoming obstacles and maintaining motivation. We will delve into the psychological theories underpinning mindset and behavior change, providing you with a toolkit of techniques to master your fitness mindset.

This eBook is designed to be interactive, featuring exercises, reflection questions, and action plans to help you apply what you learn directly to your fitness journey. By the end of this eBook, you will not only have a deeper understanding of the role mindset plays in fitness but also a personalized roadmap to achieving your fitness goals with a resilient and positive mindset.

Embarking on Your Journey

Your journey to mastering the mindset for fitness success begins now. As you turn each page, keep an open mind, be ready to challenge your existing beliefs, and prepare to transform not just your fitness, but your life. Let's embark on this journey together, with determination, resilience, and an unwavering belief in our ability to achieve greatness.

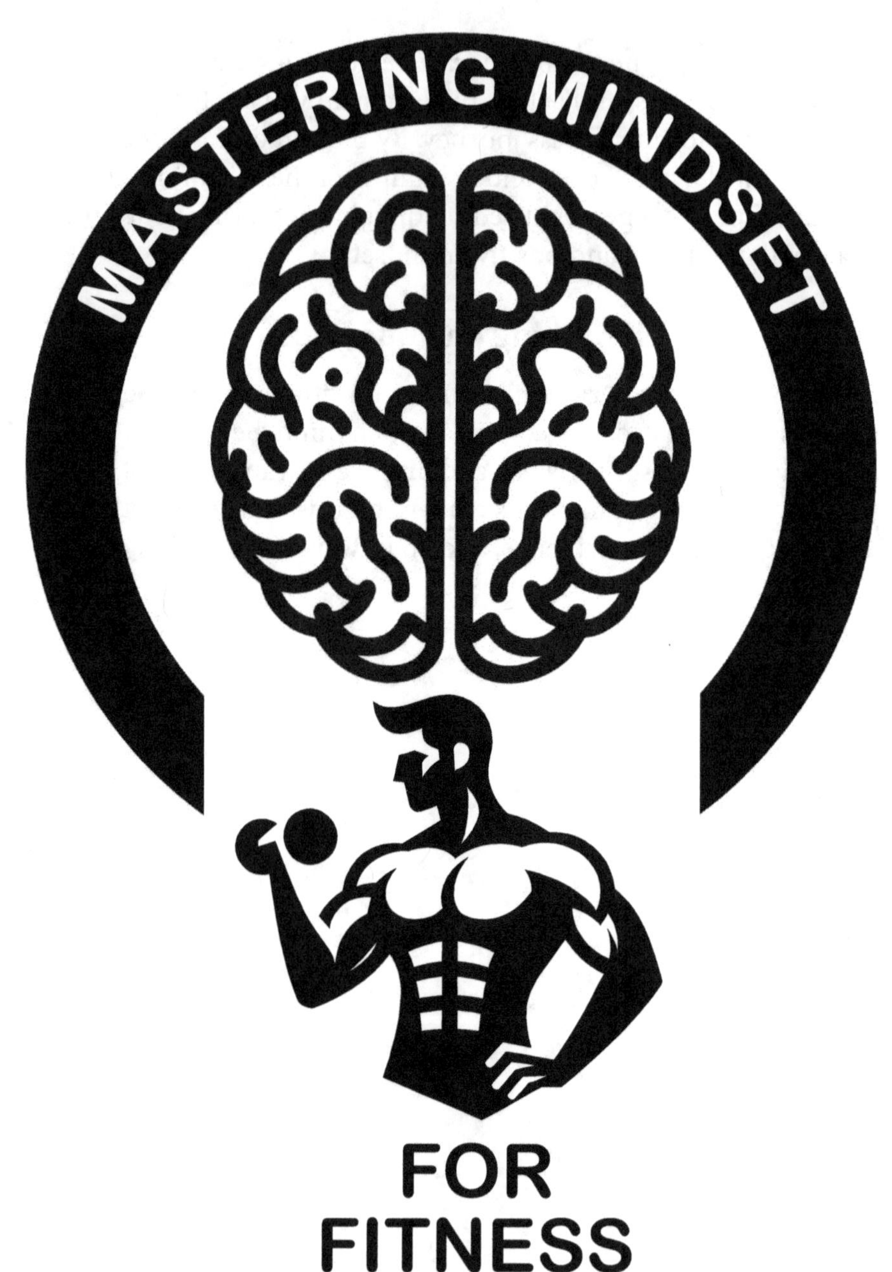

MASTERING MINDSET
FOR
FITNESS
SUCCESS

CHAPTER 2: UNDERSTANDING MINDSET

The Power of Mindset in Shaping Reality

The journey toward fitness success is as much about cultivating a resilient and positive mind as it is about honing the body. This chapter delves into the core concepts of mindset and its profound impact on our fitness endeavors. Understanding the dynamics of mindset offers the first step towards mastering it, enabling a more effective and fulfilling path to achieving your fitness goals.

Fixed vs. Growth Mindset

Central to our understanding of mindset in fitness is the distinction between a fixed mindset and a growth mindset, a concept popularized by psychologist Carol Dweck. These mindsets represent fundamentally different beliefs about learning and intelligence.

- **Fixed Mindset:** Individuals with a fixed mindset believe their abilities, intelligence, and talents are static traits. They perceive challenges as threats to their competence, often leading to avoidance of challenges and a fear of failure.

- **Growth Mindset:** In contrast, those with a growth mindset understand that their abilities and intelligence can be developed through dedication, hard work, and perseverance. They view challenges as opportunities to grow and learn, leading to greater resilience and a willingness to persist in the face of difficulties.

The Relevance of a Growth Mindset in Fitness

Adopting a growth mindset is particularly crucial in the realm of fitness, where progress is often nonlinear and fraught with setbacks. A growth mindset empowers you to:

- **Embrace Challenges:** View each new exercise, routine, or goal as an opportunity to improve, rather than an insurmountable obstacle.

- **Persist in the Face of Setbacks:** Understand that setbacks are part of the learning process, not a reflection of your inability to succeed.

- **See Effort as a Pathway to Mastery:** Recognize that consistent effort and dedication are key to improving fitness levels and achieving your goals.

- **Learn from Feedback:** Use constructive criticism as a valuable source of information for improving your fitness strategies and techniques.

Cultivating a Growth Mindset

Transitioning from a fixed to a growth mindset requires conscious effort and practice. Here are some strategies to cultivate a growth mindset in your fitness journey:

1. **Acknowledge Your Beliefs:** Become aware of your own mindset. Recognize when you are viewing challenges through a fixed mindset lens and consciously choose to

adopt a growth perspective.

2. **Embrace Challenges:** Step out of your comfort zone and embrace new fitness challenges. See them as opportunities to improve and learn, rather than threats.

3. **Celebrate Effort, Not Just Outcome:** Shift your focus from immediate results to the effort you're putting in. Progress in fitness often comes slowly; valuing effort encourages persistence.

4. **Learn from Setbacks:** Instead of getting discouraged by setbacks, analyze them to understand what went wrong and how you can improve in the future.

5. **Use Positive Self-Talk:** Challenge and replace negative thoughts with positive affirmations that reinforce your ability to grow and improve.

Conclusion

Understanding and embracing the concept of a growth mindset is a critical step in your fitness journey. It lays the foundation for resilience, motivation, and sustained effort towards achieving your fitness goals. As we move forward, keep the principles of the growth mindset at the forefront of your mind, ready to apply them to the challenges and opportunities that lie ahead in your journey to fitness success.

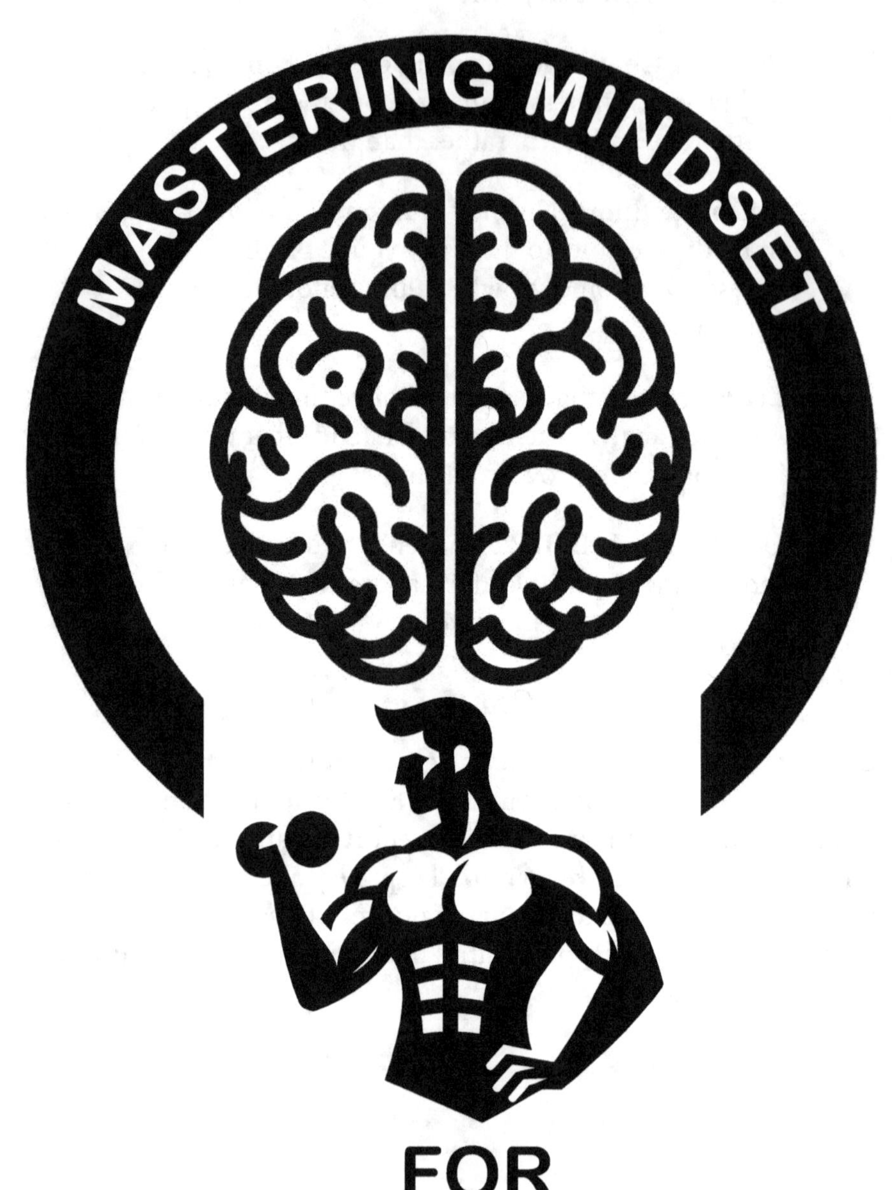

MASTERING MINDSET
FOR
FITNESS
SUCCESS

CHAPTER 3: GOAL SETTING FOR SUCCESS

The Significance of Goal Setting in Fitness

Setting well-defined, achievable goals is a cornerstone of success in any fitness journey. Goals provide direction, motivation, and a benchmark for measuring progress. This chapter focuses on the art and science of setting effective fitness goals that not only inspire action but also encourage persistence and resilience.

SMART Goals: A Framework for Success

The SMART framework is a powerful tool for setting and achieving fitness goals. SMART stands for Specific, Measurable, Achievable, Relevant, and Time-bound, each of which adds a critical layer to the goal-setting process.

- **Specific:** Goals should be clear and specific to avoid confusion about what you're trying to achieve. For example, "run a 5K" is more specific than "get fit."

- **Measurable:** Include precise amounts, dates, and so on in your goals so you can measure your degree of success. If your goal is measurable, you'll know exactly when you have achieved it.

- **Achievable:** Ensure that your goal is realistic and attainable to avoid setting yourself up for failure. It should challenge you but also be within reach.

- **Relevant:** Your goal should be important to you and align with your other objectives. A relevant goal will motivate you to commit to the effort required to achieve it.

- **Time-bound:** Your goal should have a deadline to prevent endless procrastination. Time constraints create a sense of urgency and prompt action.

Visualization and Affirmations

Beyond setting SMART goals, visualization and affirmations can significantly boost your chances of success. Visualization involves creating a vivid mental image of achieving your fitness goals, engaging all your senses to enhance the experience. This technique helps solidify your commitment and enhances motivation by enabling you to "experience" the benefits of success in advance.

Affirmations are positive, empowering statements that you repeat to yourself to overcome negative thoughts and doubts. They can reinforce your confidence and belief in your ability to achieve your goals. For example, affirming "I am capable of reaching my fitness milestones" can help maintain a positive mindset.

Setting and Pursuing Your Goals

1. **Define Your Vision:** Start with a broad vision of what you want to achieve in your fitness journey. This could be improving health, running a marathon, or achieving a certain body composition.

2. **Break It Down:** Break down your vision into specific, actionable goals using the SMART criteria. Ensure each goal aligns with your ultimate vision.

3. **Create a Plan:** For each goal, develop a plan outlining the steps needed to achieve it. Include milestones to track progress along the way.

4. **Use Visualization and Affirmations:** Regularly visualize yourself achieving your goals and use affirmations to reinforce your commitment and overcome challenges.

5. **Review and Adjust:** Regularly review your goals and progress. Be prepared to adjust your plan as needed to stay on track towards your vision.

Conclusion

Effective goal setting is a dynamic process that requires reflection, adjustment, and persistence. By setting SMART goals, employing visualization and affirmations, and actively pursuing your objectives, you can significantly enhance your motivation and resilience on the path to fitness success. As you move forward, remember that each goal achieved is a step closer to your ultimate vision, fueling your journey with purpose and direction.

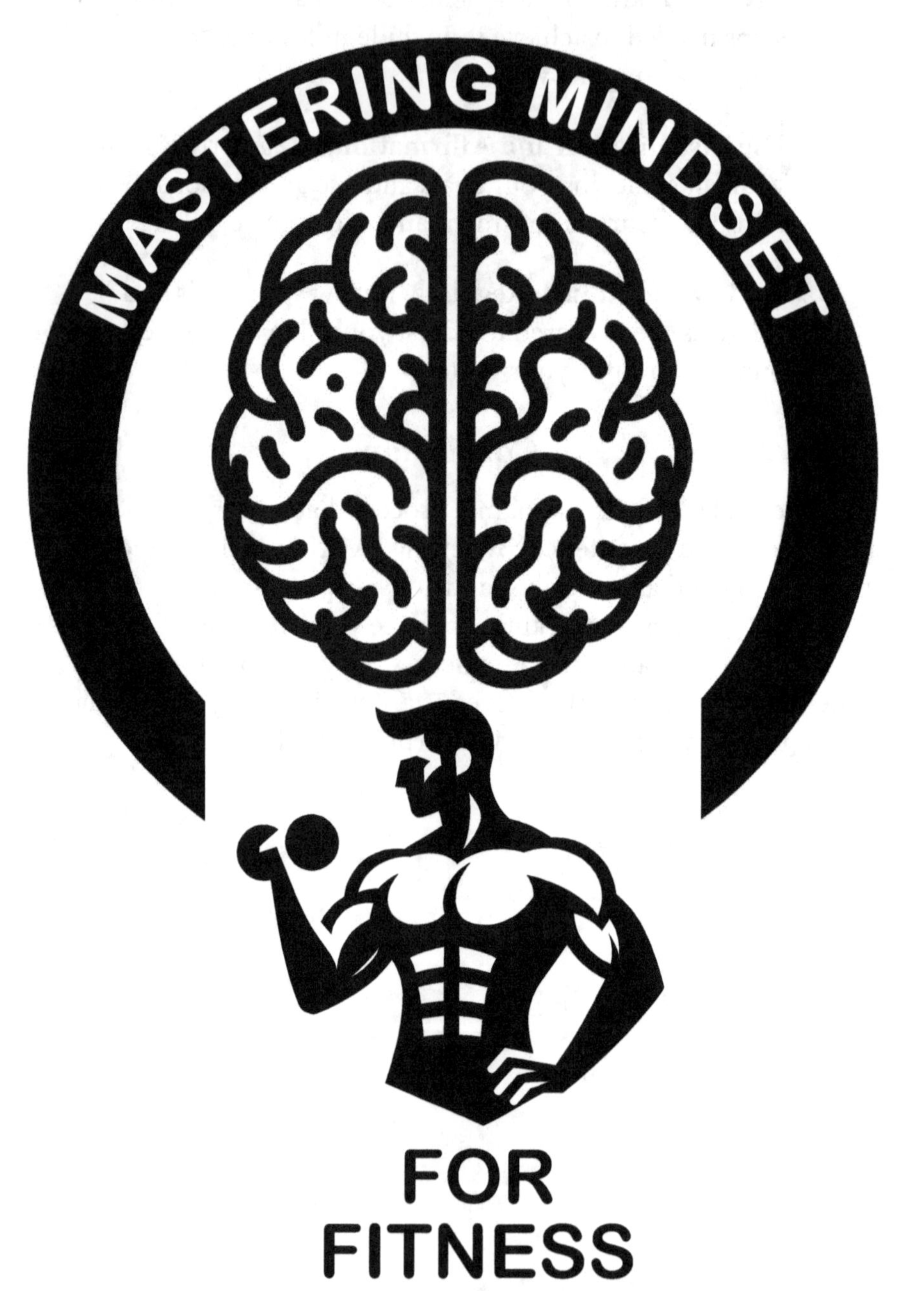
MASTERING MINDSET
FOR
FITNESS
SUCCESS

CHAPTER 4: OVERCOMING OBSTACLES

Navigating the Hurdles on Your Fitness Journey

Every fitness journey encounters obstacles. These can range from internal battles like lack of motivation or self-doubt to external challenges such as time constraints or injuries. Recognizing and overcoming these obstacles is critical to sustaining progress and achieving your fitness goals.

Identifying Common Barriers

Understanding the nature of common barriers in fitness can prepare you to tackle them effectively. Some of these include:

- **Lack of Time:** Many people struggle to fit exercise into their busy schedules.

- **Motivation Fluctuations:** Staying consistently motivated can be challenging, especially in the face of slow progress or plateaus.

- **Injuries or Physical Limitations:** Injuries can derail fitness plans, requiring modifications or rest periods.

- **Limited Resources:** Not having access to a gym, equipment, or proper nutrition can impede progress.

- **Self-Doubt:** Doubting your ability to achieve your fitness goals can be a significant mental barrier.

Strategies for Overcoming Barriers

Overcoming these obstacles requires a combination of practical strategies, mindset shifts, and sometimes, external support.

1. **Prioritize and Plan:** Address the lack of time by making fitness a priority. Schedule workouts as non-negotiable appointments in your calendar.

2. **Set Smaller, Achievable Goals:** Break down larger goals into smaller, manageable tasks to maintain motivation and a sense of progress.

3. **Adapt and Modify:** For physical limitations or injuries, consult with a healthcare provider or fitness professional to adapt your fitness plan safely.

4. **Leverage Available Resources:** Utilize free or low-cost resources, such as online workouts or outdoor activities, to overcome financial or equipment barriers.

5. **Cultivate a Supportive Community:** Engage with friends, family, or online communities for encouragement, accountability, and advice.

6. **Reframe Challenges:** Use a growth mindset to view obstacles as opportunities for learning and growth. Replace self-doubt with positive affirmations and celebrate every progress, no matter how small.

Dealing with Setbacks

Setbacks are an inevitable part of any fitness journey. The key to dealing with them effectively lies in how you respond:

- **Accept and Assess:** Recognize the setback and assess its impact objectively without self-judgment.

- **Learn from the Experience:** Identify what led to the setback and how it can inform future strategies to avoid similar obstacles.

- **Adjust Your Plan:** Make necessary adjustments to your fitness plan, whether it means setting more realistic goals, changing your approach, or incorporating new strategies to overcome the obstacle.

- **Recommit to Your Goals:** Refocus on your motivation and the reasons behind your fitness journey. Remind yourself of your ability to overcome challenges and continue moving forward.

Conclusion

Overcoming obstacles on your fitness journey is not just about finding immediate solutions but also about building resilience and adaptability. By recognizing common barriers and employing strategies to navigate them, you can maintain momentum towards your fitness goals, even in the face of challenges. Remember, each obstacle overcome is a testament to your strength, determination, and commitment to your fitness success.

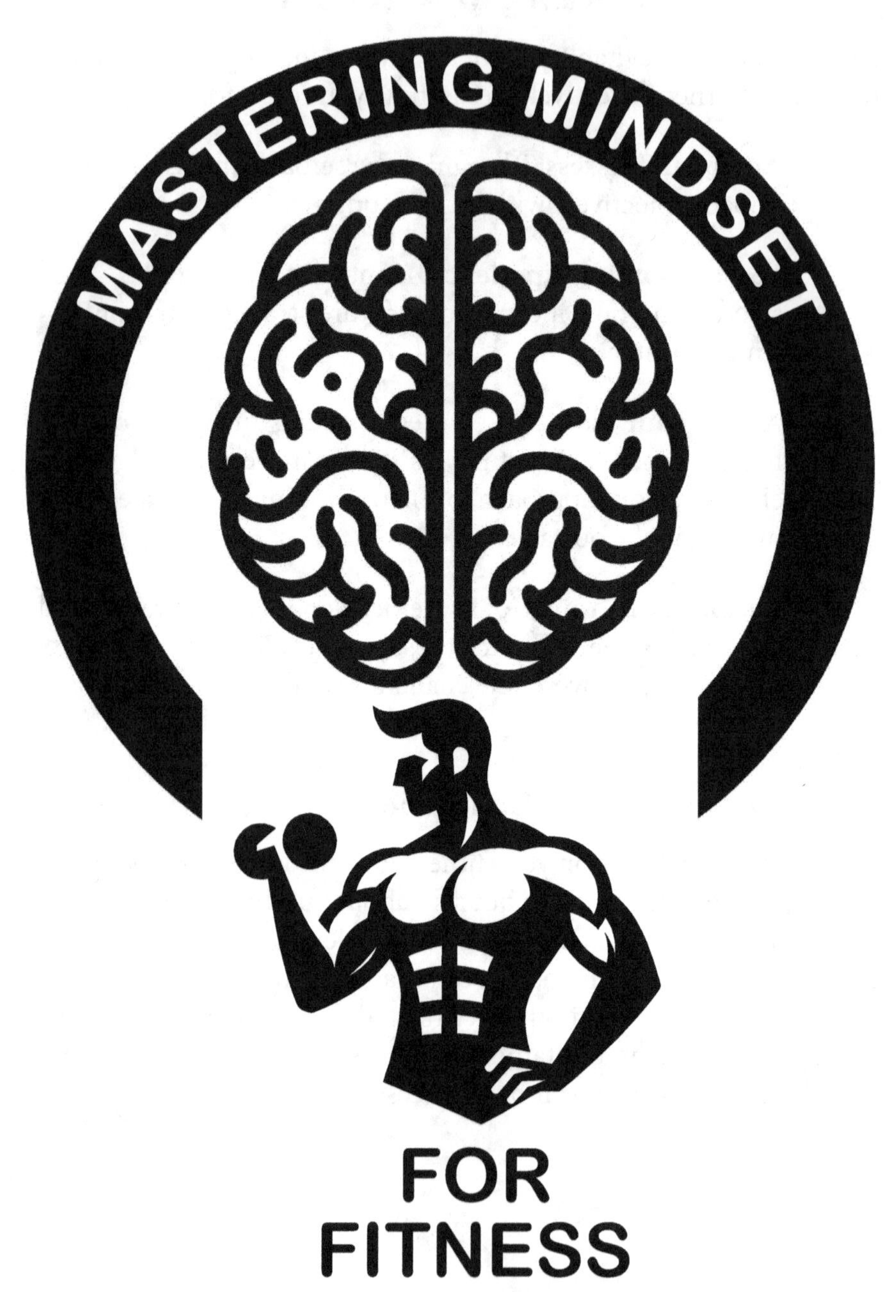

MASTERING MINDSET
FOR
FITNESS
SUCCESS

CHAPTER 5: BUILDING AND MAINTAINING MOTIVATION

The Engine of Your Fitness Journey

Motivation is the driving force behind every fitness endeavor. It initiates your journey, propels you through challenges, and sustains your commitment over time. However, maintaining motivation can be as challenging as the workouts themselves. This chapter explores strategies for building and nurturing a resilient motivational foundation.

Understanding Motivation

Motivation is not monolithic; it varies in source and intensity among individuals. It's helpful to distinguish between two primary types:

- **Intrinsic Motivation:** Comes from within and is driven by personal satisfaction or the joy of engaging in the activity itself.

- **Extrinsic Motivation:** Driven by external rewards or pressures, such as physical appearance improvements, social recognition, or competition.

Finding Your 'Why'

Identifying your core reason for pursuing fitness is crucial. Your 'why' should be compelling and personal, acting as a constant reminder of the value of your fitness journey, especially during moments of doubt or difficulty. To discover your 'why,' consider what initially inspired you to start, what you hope to achieve, and how fitness aligns with your broader life goals.

Creating a Support System

A robust support system can significantly enhance your motivation. This can include:

- **Friends and Family:** Share your goals with them and invite them to support your journey.

- **Fitness Communities:** Join online forums, social media groups, or local clubs where members share similar goals.

- **Professional Support:** Consider working with a personal trainer or coach who can provide personalized guidance and accountability.

Strategies for Sustaining Motivation

1. **Set Realistic Goals:** Use the SMART framework to set achievable goals that fuel motivation with each success.

2. **Track Progress:** Keep a log of your workouts, achievements, and how you feel. Seeing progress can be a powerful motivator.

3. **Celebrate Achievements:** Recognize and reward yourself for meeting goals, no matter how small.

4. **Mix It Up:** Variety in your workout routine can keep things

interesting and prevent boredom.

5. **Focus on the Process, Not Just the Outcome:** Enjoy the journey by celebrating small victories and learning from challenges.

6. **Revisit and Refresh Your Goals:** As you evolve, so should your goals. Regularly assess and adjust your goals to keep them challenging and relevant.

Dealing with Motivation Slumps

Even the most dedicated individuals can experience motivation slumps. When this happens:

- **Take a Break:** Sometimes, a short break can help rejuvenate your motivation.

- **Reflect on Your 'Why':** Remind yourself of the reasons behind your fitness journey.

- **Seek Inspiration:** Read success stories, watch motivational videos, or talk to someone who inspires you.

- **Adjust Your Approach:** If your current routine isn't inspiring, change it up. Try new activities that excite you.

Conclusion

Building and maintaining motivation is a dynamic and personal process. By understanding what drives you, leveraging your support system, and employing strategies to keep your motivation alive, you can navigate the ups and downs of your fitness journey with resilience and determination. Remember, the key to sustained motivation lies in connecting with your deeper purpose, celebrating your progress, and always striving towards becoming the best version of yourself.

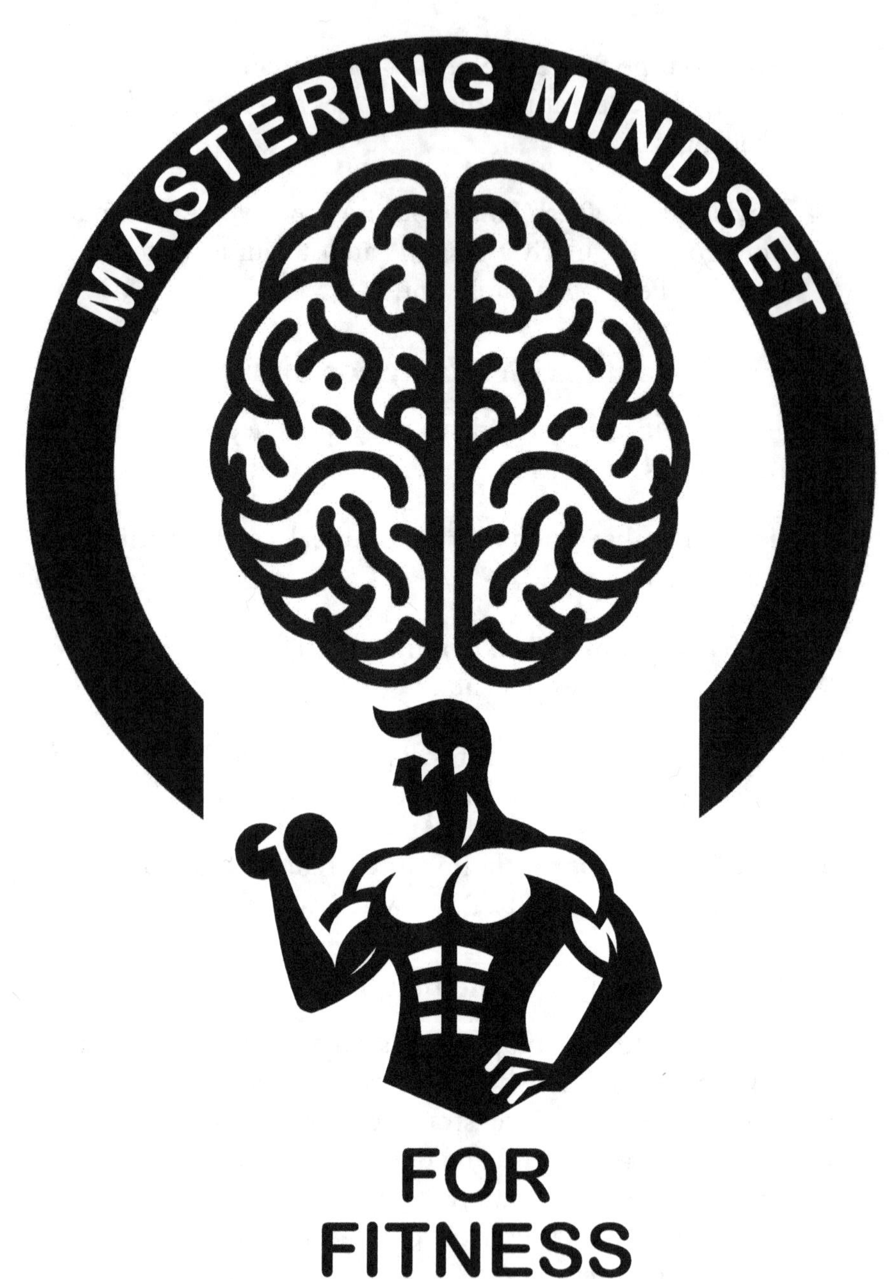

MASTERING MINDSET
FOR
FITNESS
SUCCESS

CHAPTER 6: HABIT FORMATION AND SUSTAINABILITY

Laying the Foundations for Long-term Success

Achieving fitness success is not only about making temporary changes but also about integrating those changes into your lifestyle permanently. This chapter explores how to transform fitness activities from sporadic efforts into enduring habits that contribute to long-term health and wellness.

Understanding Habit Formation

Habits are actions we perform automatically in response to a cue, without the need for deliberate decision-making. The process of habit formation involves three key components:

1. **Cue:** A trigger that initiates the behavior.

2. **Routine:** The behavior or action you want to turn into a habit.

3. **Reward:** A positive reinforcement that follows the behavior

Creating sustainable fitness habits involves identifying the right cues and rewards to make your fitness routines automatic and enjoyable.

Strategies for Building Fitness Habits

1. **Start Small:** Begin with small, manageable changes that can be easily integrated into your daily routine.

2. **Create a Cue:** Establish a consistent cue for your fitness activity, such as exercising at the same time each day or after a specific trigger like waking up.

3. **Stack Your Habits:** Link a new fitness habit with an established routine, such as doing a quick workout after your morning coffee.

4. **Focus on the Reward:** Identify immediate rewards that follow your fitness activities, like the feeling of accomplishment or a refreshing shower.

5. **Be Consistent:** Consistency is key in habit formation. Aim to perform the new behavior regularly to strengthen the habit loop.

6. **Track Your Progress:** Use a habit tracker or journal to monitor your consistency and progress, reinforcing your commitment.

7. **Be Patient and Flexible:** Building new habits takes time and may require adjustments along the way. Be patient with yourself and willing to modify your approach as needed.

Overcoming Barriers to Habit Formation

Despite the best intentions, you may encounter challenges in establishing new fitness habits. Common barriers include lack of time, loss of motivation, or external disruptions. To overcome these, consider:

- **Adjusting Your Expectations:** Recognize that perfection is not the goal; consistency is. It's okay to miss a day or adjust your habits as needed.

- **Finding Alternative Solutions:** If time is a constraint, look for ways to incorporate more efficient workouts into your day or combine activities.

- **Seeking Support:** Use your support system to stay accountable and motivated.

Making Fitness a Sustainable Part of Your Life

Sustainability in fitness means making choices and establishing habits that you can maintain over the long haul. It involves balancing effort with enjoyment, pushing for progress while also allowing for rest and recovery.

1. **Listen to Your Body:** Pay attention to your body's signals. Rest when needed and avoid pushing through pain or fatigue.

2. **Incorporate Variety:** Keep your fitness routine engaging by trying new activities, workouts, and challenges.

3. **Adjust Goals Over Time:** As you grow and change, your fitness goals should evolve too. Regularly reassess and adjust your goals to reflect your current aspirations and abilities.

Conclusion

The transformation of fitness activities into lasting habits is essential for long-term success. By understanding the mechanics of habit formation and employing effective strategies, you can make fitness a natural and enjoyable part of your daily life. Remember, the goal is not only to achieve immediate fitness outcomes but to cultivate a lifestyle that promotes continuous growth, health, and well-being.

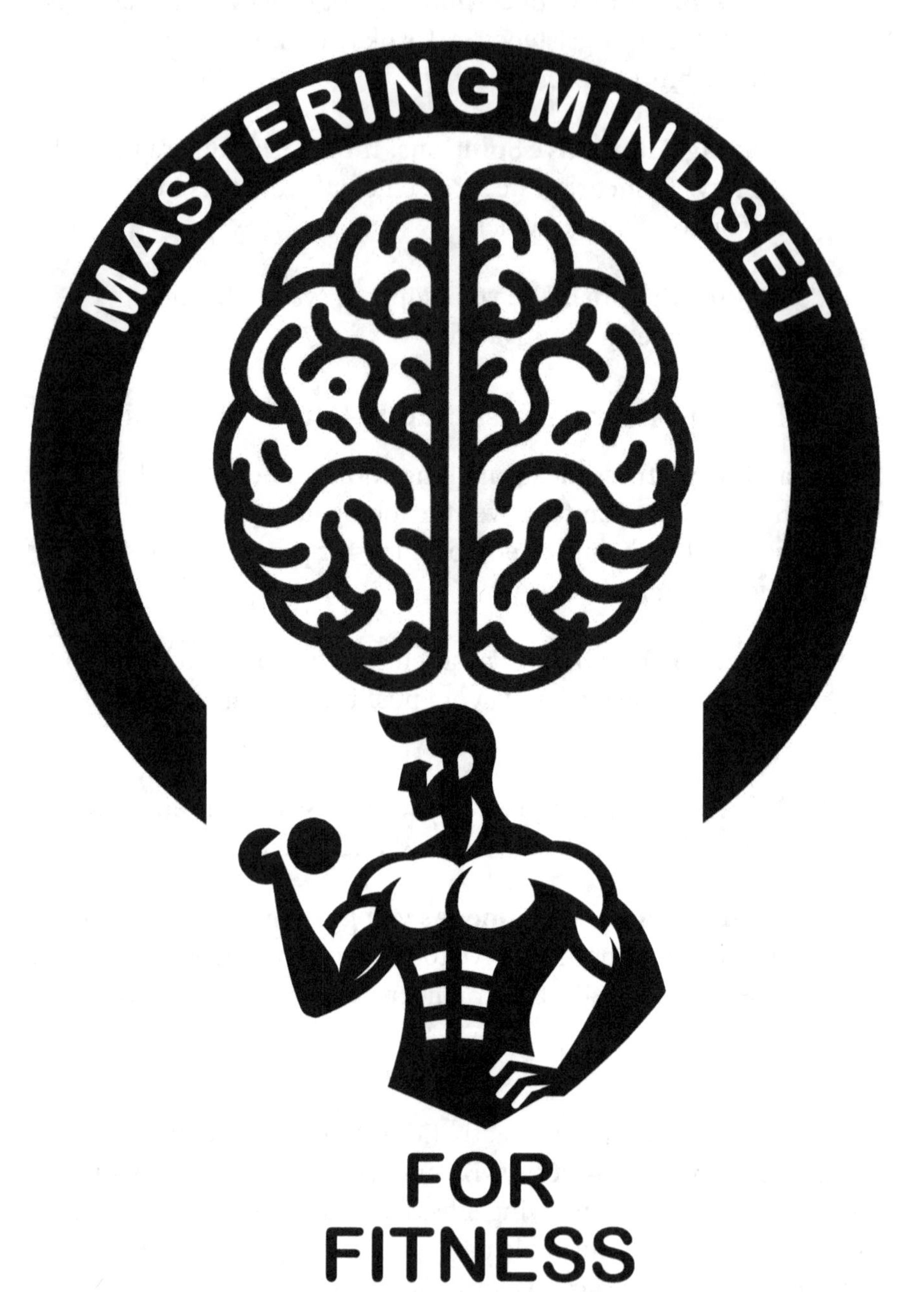

MASTERING MINDSET
FOR
FITNESS
SUCCESS

CHAPTER 7: ADVANCED MINDSET MASTERY

Elevating Your Fitness Journey Through Mindfulness and NLP

As you progress on your fitness journey, mastering your mindset becomes increasingly important. Advanced techniques like mindfulness and Neuro-Linguistic Programming (NLP) can provide you with the tools to navigate challenges, enhance focus, and achieve a deeper sense of motivation and satisfaction. This chapter explores how these techniques can be integrated into your fitness routine to foster a more profound connection between mind and body, leading to greater overall success.

Mindfulness in Fitness

Mindfulness involves maintaining a moment-by-moment awareness of our thoughts, feelings, bodily sensations, and surrounding environment. It encourages a non-judgmental acceptance of our present experience.

1. **Benefits in Fitness:**

- **Enhanced Focus:** Mindfulness helps improve concentration and focus during workouts, allowing for better technique and performance.

- **Stress Reduction:** Regular mindfulness practice can reduce stress, which can otherwise hinder recovery and performance.

Improved Body Awareness: Being mindful enhances body awareness, helping you recognize when to push harder and when to pull back to prevent injury.

2. **Practical Applications:**

- **Mindful Breathing:** Before beginning your workout, spend a few minutes focusing on your breath. This can center your mind, reduce pre-workout stress, and improve oxygen flow to your muscles.

- **Mindful Movement:** Pay attention to each movement during your workout, noticing the sensations in your muscles and the rhythm of your breath. This can enhance the mind-body connection and increase the effectiveness of your workout.

Neuro-Linguistic Programming (NLP)

NLP is a psychological approach that involves analyzing strategies used by successful individuals and applying them to reach a personal goal. It relates to understanding and harnessing the power of language to change our patterns of mental behavior and achieve specific outcomes.

1. **Benefits in Fitness:**

- **Reframing Thoughts:** NLP teaches how to change negative thought patterns into positive ones, which can be especially useful for overcoming mental barriers to fitness success.

- **Setting Clear Goals:** The clarity and precision in goal-setting advocated by NLP can lead to more effective and achievable fitness targets.

- **Enhancing Motivation:** NLP techniques can help identify what truly motivates you, tapping into deeper sources of motivation beyond surface-level desires.

2.　**Practical Applications:**

- **Visualizing Success:** Use NLP visualization techniques to create a clear, compelling image of your fitness goals, including how achieving them will look, sound, and feel. This can significantly enhance motivation and commitment.

- **Positive Self-Talk:** Adopt NLP methods to transform your internal dialogue. Replace self-critical or doubting thoughts with empowering affirmations that support your fitness journey.

Integrating Mindfulness and NLP into Your Fitness Routine

Combining mindfulness and NLP techniques can supercharge your fitness journey, offering a robust toolkit for overcoming mental challenges and enhancing physical performance. Here are some ways to integrate these approaches:

- **Begin Each Day with Intention:** Use mindfulness to set a focused intention for your day and NLP to frame it in positive, empowering language.

- **Incorporate Mindful Moments:** Throughout your day and during workouts, take brief moments to practice mindfulness, reconnecting with your body and breath.

- **Use NLP for Goal Setting:** Apply NLP techniques when setting fitness goals, ensuring they are clear, positive, and aligned with your deeper motivations.

Conclusion

Mastering advanced mindset techniques like mindfulness and NLP can transform your approach to fitness, offering deeper insights into your motivations, enhancing your focus and performance, and helping you navigate the psychological challenges of a fitness journey. By incorporating these practices, you empower yourself to achieve not only your fitness goals but also a greater sense of well-being and fulfillment.

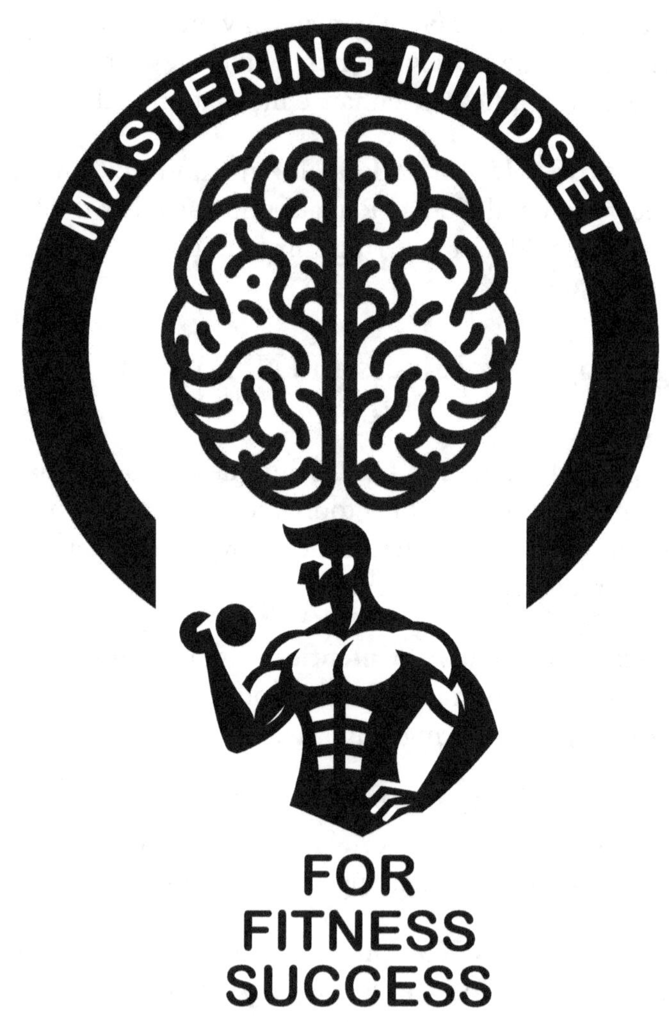

CHAPTER 8: SUCCESS STORIES

Inspiration Through Transformation

One of the most compelling ways to motivate and encourage individuals on their fitness journey is through the power of success stories. These narratives not only provide tangible proof of what's possible but also offer insights into the diverse strategies individuals employ to overcome challenges and achieve their fitness goals. In this chapter, we'll share a series of success stories that highlight the critical role of mindset in achieving fitness success.

Story 1: The Marathon Runner

Background: John, a 40-year-old with no prior running experience, set a goal to complete a marathon within a year. Initially overwhelmed by the magnitude of his challenge, he focused on cultivating a growth mindset, setting small, achievable milestones, and gradually increasing his endurance and confidence.

Strategies for Success:

- **SMART Goal Setting:** John began with short runs, progressively increasing his distance each week.

- **Overcoming Obstacles:** He dealt with several injuries by consulting professionals, adjusting his training, and focusing on recovery.

- **Mindset Mastery:** John used visualization techniques to imagine himself crossing the finish line, which kept him motivated during tough times.

Outcome: After a year of dedicated training, John completed his first marathon, surpassing his own expectations and inspiring others to pursue their fitness goals.

Story 2: The Weight Loss Journey

Background: Sarah, a 35-year-old mother of two, aimed to lose 50 pounds and improve her overall health. Facing time constraints and initial lack of motivation, Sarah embraced a positive mindset, focusing on the benefits her fitness journey would bring to her and her family.

Strategies for Success:

- **Building Habits:** Sarah incorporated 30 minutes of exercise into her daily routine, finding activities she enjoyed to ensure consistency.

- **Nutritional Awareness:** She educated herself on nutrition, making healthier food choices that supported her weight loss goals.

- **Support System:** Sarah joined a fitness group with similar goals for motivation and accountability.

Outcome: Over 18 months, Sarah reached her weight loss target and significantly improved her physical and mental health. Her story became a source of inspiration for her community.

Story 3: The Strength Transformation

Background: Alex, a 25-year-old software developer, wanted to build strength and muscle. Initially struggling with self-doubt and inconsistency, Alex adopted a growth mindset, focusing on progress over perfection and celebrating each small victory.

Strategies for Success:

- **Consistent Training:** Alex committed to a structured strength training program, tracking his workouts and progress.

- **Learning and Adaptation:** He invested time in learning proper techniques and nutrition, adjusting his plan based on results and feedback.

- **Mindful Reflection:** Alex used mindfulness to stay present during workouts and reflect on his progress, reinforcing his commitment to his goals.

Outcome: Within two years, Alex transformed his physique, gaining significant muscle mass and strength. His journey underscored the importance of patience, perseverance, and a positive mindset.

Conclusion

These success stories exemplify the transformative power of a positive mindset in achieving fitness goals. Each individual faced unique challenges but through a combination of strategic goal setting, overcoming obstacles, and mindset mastery, they were able to achieve remarkable results. Let these stories inspire you to believe in your potential and embark on your own journey of fitness success with confidence and determination.

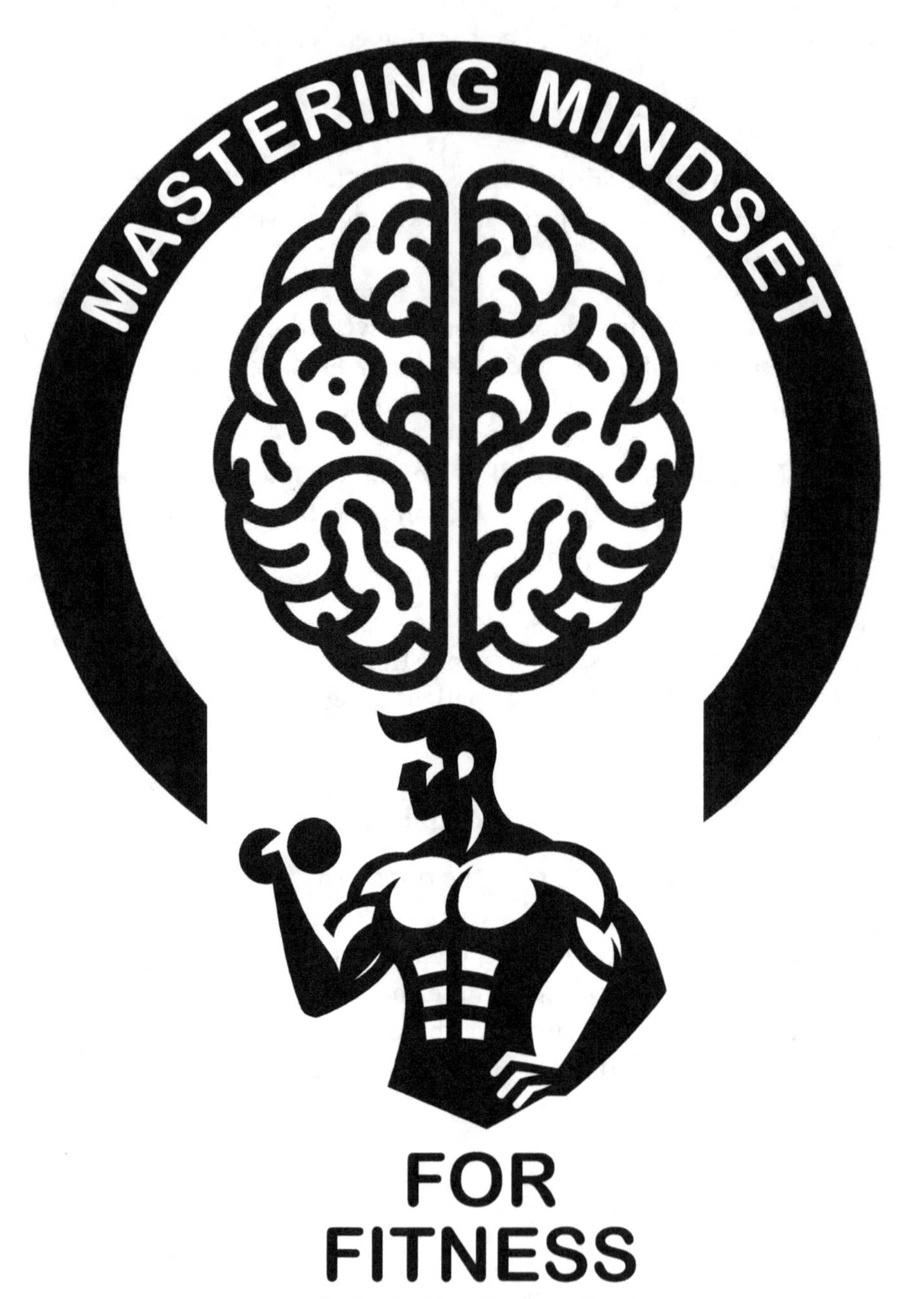

MASTERING MINDSET
FOR
FITNESS
SUCCESS

CHAPTER 9: PUTTING IT ALL TOGETHER

Crafting Your Personalized Action Plan

Having explored the essential elements of cultivating a positive mindset, setting and achieving goals, overcoming obstacles, maintaining motivation, forming sustainable habits, and drawing inspiration from success stories, it's now time to synthesize these insights into a personalized action plan. This chapter will guide you through developing a structured, actionable plan to apply the principles discussed to your fitness journey.

Step 1: Define Your Vision and Goals

Begin by clearly defining your overarching vision for your fitness journey. What does ultimate success look like to you? Use the SMART criteria to set specific, measurable, achievable, relevant, and time-bound goals that align with this vision. Ensure your goals are motivated by a deep 'why' that resonates with your values and aspirations.

Step 2: Assess and Prepare

Take stock of your current situation, including your strengths, areas for improvement, and any potential obstacles. Preparation involves planning how to leverage your strengths and address weaknesses. This may include gathering resources, seeking knowledge, or creating a supportive environment for your journey.

Step 3: Develop a Strategy

Based on your goals and assessment, develop a comprehensive strategy that encompasses workout plans, nutrition, rest, and recovery. Incorporate techniques for mindset mastery, such as mindfulness and positive self-talk, to strengthen your mental approach. Outline specific actions, schedules, and milestones to guide your progress.

Step 4: Implement Your Plan

With your plan in place, it's time to take action. Begin implementing your strategy, focusing on consistency and adaptability. Use tools like journals or apps to track your progress, and don't hesitate to adjust your plan as you learn what works best for you.

Step 5: Monitor and Adjust

Regularly review your progress against your goals and the milestones you've set. Celebrate your successes, however small, and reflect on any setbacks, viewing them as opportunities for growth. Be prepared to make adjustments to your plan based on feedback from your body, performance, and overall well-being.

Step 6: Sustain and Evolve

As you achieve your initial goals, set new ones to continue your fitness journey. Explore new activities, techniques, and challenges to keep your routine engaging and your motivation high. Remember, fitness is a lifelong journey of growth and self-discovery.

Resources for Further Learning

Conclude your action plan with a list of resources for further learning and inspiration. This might include books, websites, apps, or communities related to fitness, nutrition, and mindset mastery. Continual learning is key to staying motivated and informed on your journey.

Conclusion

Your personalized action plan is a living document that will guide you through the complexities of your fitness journey. By putting the principles of mindset, goal setting, habit formation, and perseverance into action, you're not just working towards your fitness goals; you're cultivating a lifestyle that promotes growth, health, and happiness. Remember, the journey itself is as important as the destination. Embrace each step, stay flexible, and celebrate your progress. You have the tools and knowledge to achieve fitness success; now, it's time to turn your vision into reality.

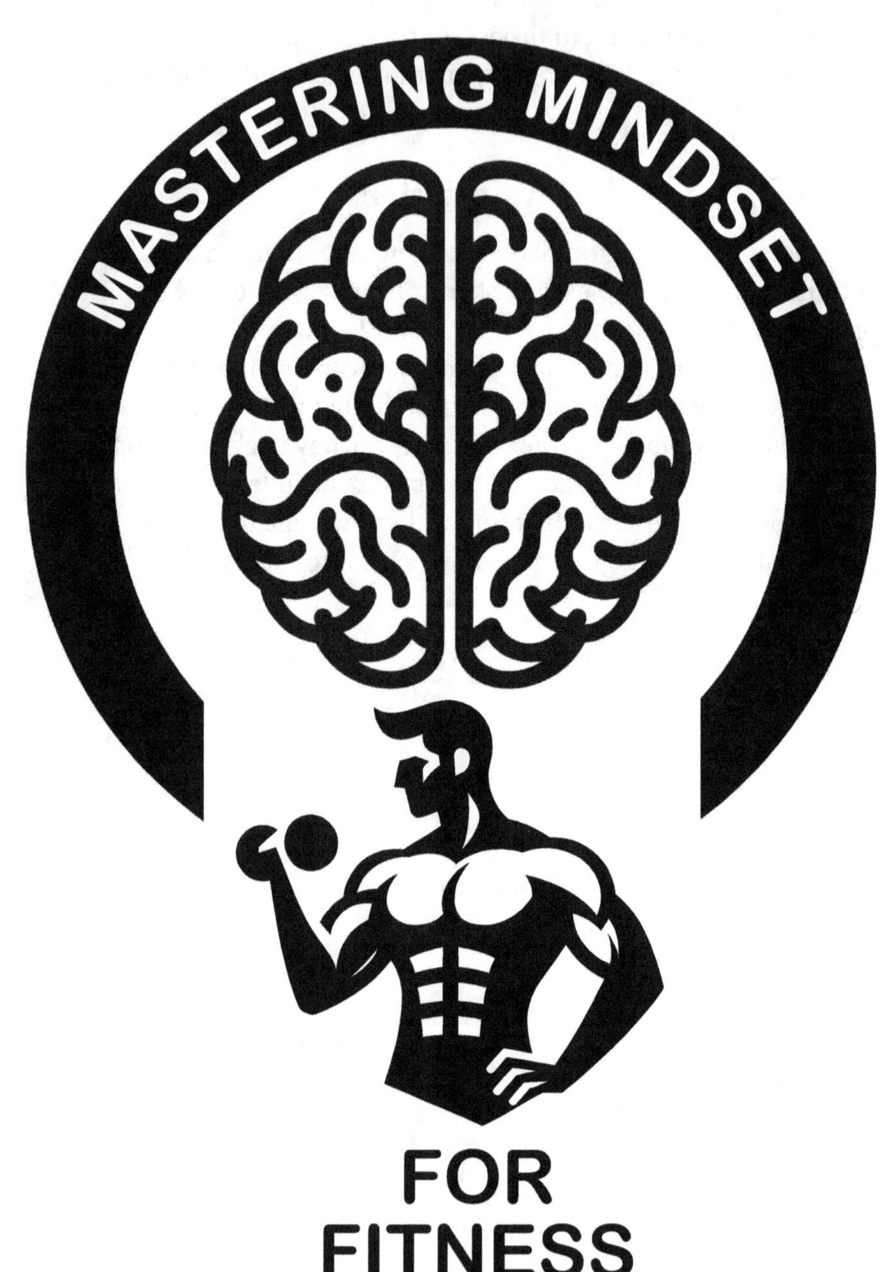

MASTERING MINDSET
FOR
FITNESS
SUCCESS

CHAPTER 10: KEY PRINCIPLES

Reflecting on the Journey Ahead

As we conclude "Mastering Mindset for Fitness Success," it's important to pause and reflect on the journey you are about to embark on or continue with renewed insight. This eBook has equipped you with the tools, strategies, and inspiration needed to cultivate a positive mindset that supports your fitness goals. Embracing the principles outlined here will not only enhance your physical health but also contribute to your overall well-being and personal growth.

Key Takeaways

- **Mindset is Fundamental:** A growth mindset is the bedrock of fitness success, empowering you to embrace challenges, learn from setbacks, and persist in the face of obstacles.

- **Goal Setting Guides the Way:** SMART goals provide a clear, actionable path toward achieving your fitness aspirations, while visualization and affirmations keep you aligned and motivated.

- **Overcoming Obstacles Builds Resilience:** Identifying

common barriers and employing strategies to overcome them strengthens your resolve and adaptability, making you more resilient.

- **Motivation Fuels Your Progress:** Understanding and nurturing your motivation, through both intrinsic and extrinsic sources, ensures sustained effort and engagement in your fitness journey.

- **Habits Anchor Your Success:** Transforming fitness activities into enduring habits is key to integrating health and wellness into your lifestyle for the long term.

- **Advanced Techniques Elevate Your Journey:** Incorporating mindfulness and NLP can deepen your connection to your fitness goals, enhancing both mental and physical performance.

- **Success Stories Inspire:** Real-life transformations underscore the power of mindset in achieving remarkable fitness goals and serve as a beacon of possibility.

Moving Forward

As you move forward, remember that the journey to fitness success is uniquely yours. It will be filled with highs and lows, triumphs and challenges. What matters most is your commitment to persist, adapt, and grow. Let the principles and strategies you've learned serve as a compass, guiding you toward your goals.

Your Fitness Success Story

Imagine, one day, sharing your own success story, not only to celebrate your achievements but also to inspire others to embark on their own journeys. Your story could be the catalyst for someone else's transformation, contributing to a cycle of positivity and growth.

Final Words of Encouragement

As you close this book and prepare to write the next chapter of your fitness journey, remember: the power to achieve your goals lies within you. The journey will require hard work, dedication, and resilience, but the rewards—improved health, confidence, and a sense of accomplishment—are immeasurable.

Stay focused on your vision, embrace the journey with an open heart and mind, and trust in your ability to achieve greatness. You have the tools, knowledge, and inspiration to master your fitness mindset and succeed. Now, it's time to take action and make your fitness dreams a reality.

Thank you for embarking on this journey through "Mastering Mindset for Fitness Success." Here's to your health, happiness, and the incredible journey ahead.

ABOUT THE AUTHOR

Adam Fraser is a renowned fitness trainer whose innovative approaches and dedication to wellness have transformed the lives of many, including celebrities like Tyler Perry. Based in California, Adam has built a career on the foundation of holistic health, emphasizing the balance between physical training, mental resilience, and nutritional guidance. With a passion for empowering individuals to achieve their highest potential, Adam has become a sought-after expert in personal transformation.

Through his work at Body Reborn Fitness, Adam offers a comprehensive approach to fitness that goes beyond traditional workouts, incorporating cutting-edge techniques and personalized strategies to ensure lasting success. His methods are informed by years of experience and a deep understanding of the intricate relationship between mind and body.

Adam is not just a trainer; he's a motivator, a mentor, and an advocate for a lifestyle that celebrates strength, flexibility, and mental clarity. His commitment to excellence and his ability to inspire has garnered a loyal following and widespread acclaim.

For more information on Adam's programs, visit http://bodyrebornfitness.com. Join our vibrant community for discussions, video courses, weekly webinar meetings, and downloadable resources at http://app.bodyrebornfitness.com.

GLOSSARY OF KEY TERMS

Aerobic Exercise: Physical activity that increases heart rate and oxygen to muscles over an extended period, improving cardiovascular health.

Anaerobic Exercise: Intense physical activity that causes lactate to form, designed to build power and muscle mass.

BMI (Body Mass Index): A measure of body fat based on height and weight that applies to adult men and women.

Core Strength: The strength of the muscles in your torso, especially your lower back and abdominal area, which are essential for stability and preventing injury.

HIIT (High-Intensity Interval Training): A training technique involving intense bursts of exercise followed by short recovery periods.

Mindfulness: The practice of being fully present and engaged in the moment, aware of your thoughts and feelings without distraction or judgment.

Nutrition: The process of providing or obtaining the food necessary for health and growth.

Recovery: The rest period essential for muscle repair, strength building, and performance enhancement following exercise.

Resistance Training: A form of exercise that improves muscular strength and endurance by doing repetitive exercises with weights, weight machines, or resistance bands.

Set: A group of repetitions of a specific exercise done without stopping.

Repetition (Rep): The completion of an exercise movement from start to finish.

TESTIMONIALS

"Adam Fraser's training program has been a game-changer for me. His personalized approach and comprehensive understanding of fitness and nutrition have helped me achieve goals I thought were out of reach. I've never felt better!"

—Tyler Perry

"Training with Adam not only transformed my body but also my mindset towards health and fitness. His methods are effective, and his motivational support is unwavering. Highly recommend Body Reborn Fitness!"

—Mary V.

"Adam's expertise and personalized fitness plans have made a significant difference in my life. His focus on holistic wellness and mental resilience alongside physical fitness is truly inspiring. I'm grateful to be part of the Body Reborn Fitness community."

—Michael R.

FREQUENTLY ASKED QUESTIONS

Q: How do I start my fitness journey with Body Reborn Fitness?

A: Visit our website at bodyrebornfitness.com to learn about our programs. Join our community at app.bodyrebornfitness.com for personalized plans.

Q: What makes Body Reborn Fitness different from other fitness programs?

A: Our holistic approach, focusing on physical fitness, mental wellness, and nutrition, tailored to each individual's needs.

Q: Can I follow the program if I have dietary restrictions?

A: Yes, our nutritional guidance is customized to accommodate dietary restrictions and preferences.

Q: How often are the weekly webinars and what do they cover?

A: Webinars are held weekly, covering a range of topics from workout techniques to mental resilience and nutritional advice.

NEXT STEPS

Take the next step in your fitness journey. Sign up for our email list or join our empowering community in the web app - accessible on all platforms. Embrace a holistic approach to wellness and become the best version of yourself with Body Reborn Fitness.

Email Sign Up:

http://bodyrebornfitness.com

Community Sign Up:

http://app.bodyrebornfitness.com

Feedback

Your feedback is invaluable to us. Share your thoughts, experiences, and suggestions to help us improve and better serve our community.

Let us know how we're doing:

http://bodyrebornfitness.com/feedback

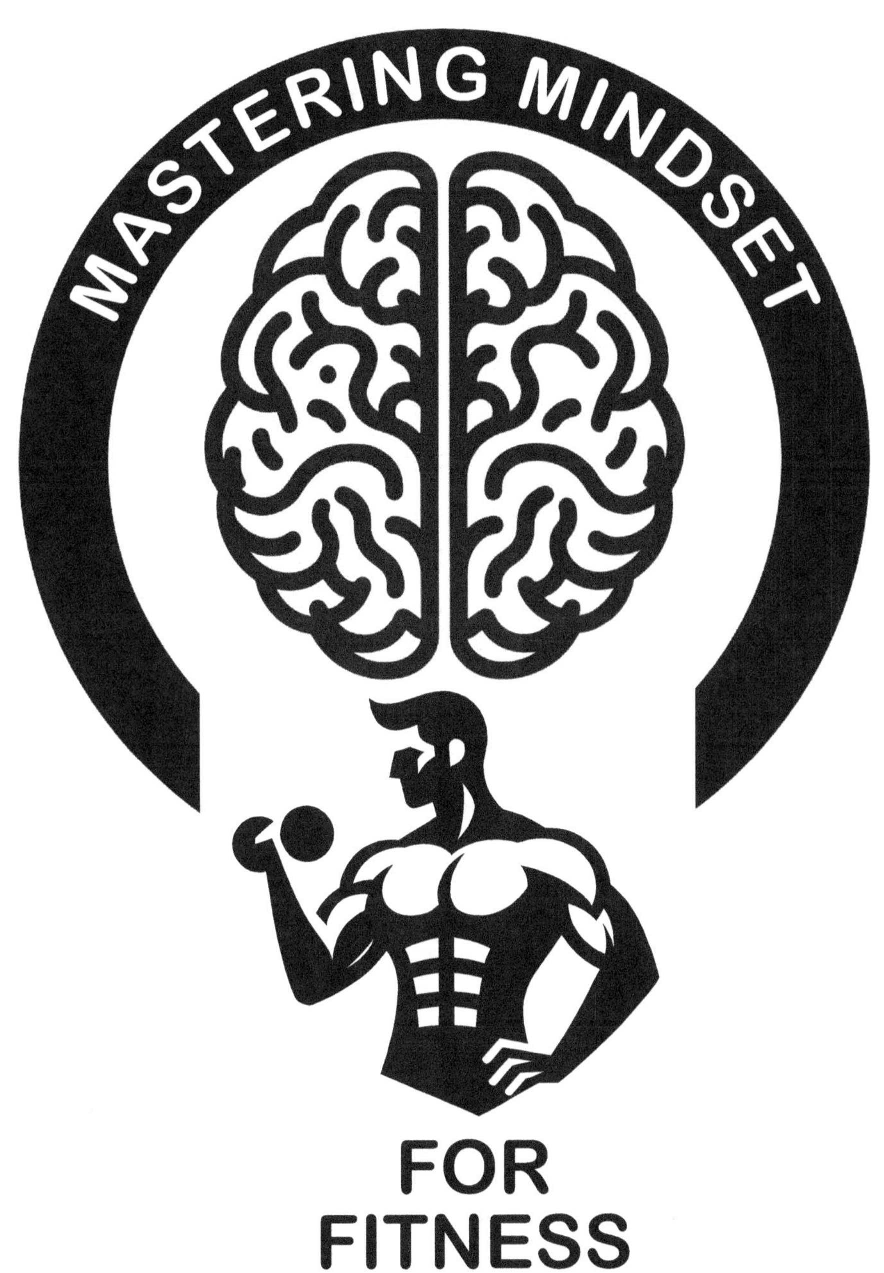

MASTERING MINDSET
FOR
FITNESS
SUCCESS